Minimalist's Guide to R

Finish Your Ultra by Tr

By Terry Gebhardt

Minimalist's Guide to Running an Ultramarathon-Finish Your Ultra by Training Smarter, Not Harder! © 2017 Terry Gebhardt

All rights reserved. No part of this book may be reproduced in any form without the permission in writing from the author.

Disclaimer

The information contained in this book is for informational purposes only. It is not intended as medical or professional advice of any kind. This book does not constitute or create a physical therapist-patient relationship. Your participation in the program in this book and viewing of the videos neither constitutes nor creates a physical therapist-patient relationship or any type of professional relationship with its author. Similarly, your voluntary viewing of the videos, participation in the program, and use of the information provided herein constitutes an assumption of the risks associated with the activities depicted therein, and your agreement to hold the author harmless from any adverse result or injury suffered by anyone.

Your Free Gift

As a way of saying thank you for your purchase, I'm offering you free access to the videos from my mini-course: 8 Simple Steps to Improving Your Running Technique.

As an ultrarunner, physical therapist, and running coach I have a unique perspective on running. My passion is helping runners improve their running performance while enabling them to run forever, injury-free. The 8 short videos in this series will help get you on your way to running stronger, injury-free!

Sign up at StrongerOverForty.com to get access to the videos and be the first to get training tips to help you run stronger!

Table of Contents

Introduction 6
Why do so many runners DNF (Did Not Finish)? 8
Can you run 100 miles? 10
How do you run strong and avoid injury? 17
How is your running technique? 21
What is the best running shoe for you? 25
Understanding common running injuries 29
Why all runners need to understand pain 33
Your nutrition and hydration plan 40
Your training plan 42
Final recommendations 57

Introduction

Why is the DNF (Did Not Finish) rate so high for ultramarathons? Depending on the race, it is not unusual to have a DNF rate of 30% or greater. What training program will give you the best chance to finish a 50 or 100-mile race? The good news is that you don't need to run as many miles as you probably think you do. In fact, running too much will put you at risk for a DNF. This book is your blueprint for finishing an ultramarathon and includes several key training pieces most runners neglect in their training. After reading this book, you will understand why the DNF rate is so high. More importantly, you will have the exact elements of a perfect training program so you can be confident you will finish your ultramarathon.

The sport of ultrarunning has seen tremendous growth over the last several years. Many runners are finding the physical and mental challenges of a 50 or 100-mile race provides a huge sense of accomplishment. I got into the sport for the physical and mental challenge, not because I love to run. I didn't grow up being a runner. I ran a few marathons in college when 26.2 miles seemed like a long distance (again, mostly for the mental and physical challenge). After undergrad, I went on to physical therapy school and was a physical therapist in the Army for 8 years. I continued recreational running (<15 miles per week) and did some adventure racing when I was in the military. When I got out of the Army, I moved to Colorado and the Pike's Peak Ascent Half Marathon caught my attention. I was intrigued by the challenge of doing a half marathon uphill. Following that race, I needed another challenge. That is when I learned about the sport of ultrarunning. I set my goal to run the Leadville 100 the following Summer so I could qualify for the Hardrock 100. I finished Leadville only 13 minutes before the cut off time. Two years later I completed the Hardrock 100.

My reason for telling you my story is to help you understand and more importantly help you believe you can finish an ultramarathon without it taking over your life (unless you want it to). You can run an ultra and not battle injuries throughout your training. You just need a system that tells you exactly what to do. Trust the process, follow your training plan, and you will finish your next ultramarathon!

Why do so many runners DNF (Did Not Finish)?

Let's dig deeper into why the DNF rate is so high? There can be many reasons, but one of the main reasons is overtraining. Many runners, especially ones addicted to running, feel more training is better. More training is not better training. Smarter training is better training. Many runners put in high mileage weeks and don't give themselves enough recovery. It is important to remember that your body gets stronger during your recovery time. If you don't allow enough recovery time, you are setting yourself up for injury. You can get away with not allowing enough recovery time for a while, but eventually it will catch up with you. Unfortunately, this often happens when runners are pushing themselves during a race leading to a DNF.

Recovery is important for more than just your muscles, tendons, and joints. Your whole body is stressed when you run. It needs time to recover and get stronger as well. Many runners can be plagued by nausea and vomiting during an ultramarathon. Many factors can cause nausea. High altitude, not eating or drinking enough, or eating or drinking too much are some of the most common causes. However, many runners don't consider how the stress of race day affects their gut. Have you ever had "butterflies" before a race? Or to be cruder...have you ever had a "nervous poo" before a race? Some runners experience no GI (gastrointestinal) issues during training, but consistently experience them on race day. The stress of a race day, even if it's a good stress, can be just enough to trigger nausea when combined with all the other factors. When I was training for the

Hardrock 100, there were many times I had a "nervous poo" just thinking about the race. Talk about stress!

Another major factor contributing to the high DNF rate is not training mentally. Mental training is much more than being able to push yourself when you get tired. Going into a race, every runner must realize and expect life will suck at some point (or many points) during the race. A strong mental training program will help you work through these moments. There was a time during the San Juan Solstice 50 mile race when I felt nauseous and vomited for 2-3 hours during the race. I was unable to eat or drink much and couldn't run. I worked through this part the of race and finished feeling incredibly strong ditching my pacer during the last mile of the race! The mental tactics you will learn in this book will give you the confidence you need to succeed.

Can you run 100 miles?

Before you register for any ultramarathon you need to be certain you can and will finish the race. You may be thinking "anything can happen on race day regardless of how well I train and how much I believe I will finish". Of course, there will be things on race day you cannot control. However, the more prepared you are mentally to deal with these things, the more likely you will be able to overcome them and finish the race. If you have even a small doubt about your ability to finish the race, that uncertainty will become much greater when you encounter your first setback during the race.

The first step is to either not look at the DNF number or if you do, don't let it psych you out. Many first-time ultra-runners look at the DNF number or talk to other runners who DNFed (did not finish). Don't let what other runners failed to do affect your confidence. I made this mistake when I was training for the Leadville 100. An elite level cyclist and very respectable runner told me how he had attempted the Leadville 100 twice and did not finish. The first thing that went through my mind was, "if he couldn't do this, how am I going to especially when the longest race I've ever done has been a marathon?". I had similar thoughts looking at the DNF list from years past. I would see the same names several years in a row and think these runners have tried 2 or 3 times (sometimes more) and still haven't finished. Don't give yourself an easy out and make it OK to DNF before you even start the race. It is important to focus on yourself and your training program. Remember why most runners DNF and know your training program will include everything you need to give you the best possible chance of success. It does however, require hard work, discipline, and following a plan.

Your Mental Performance Training Program

Can you develop your mental toughness? Absolutely! A key part of your training is to "get comfortable being uncomfortable". There will be times during the race when you will feel like crap. You may be cold, tired, hot, nauseous, have blisters, or maybe just want to cry. You will hear that voice in your head that remembers the DNF rate or the other runners you talked to who DNFed. That voice will justify quitting by thinking "I'm doing great just to try this" or "I can try again next year", or "it takes some runners 3 times to finish an ultra and this is only my first". It is OK to have these thoughts. However, you must be able to work through them and push on. Practicing being uncomfortable is an important part of your training program. A key part of your practice is to learn how to smile and "embrace the suck". This means training yourself to simply smile and enjoy the moment knowing it will pass. Many successful ultra-runners have this mentality already. If you do, you are well on your way to a solid finish. The good news is you can train yourself to feel that way. Your reality is what your brain creates. If you think something is going to suck, it will. If you think "I love this, I feel strong, I feel great", you will!

Here are some things you can do to practice being uncomfortable:

- Take a cold shower or make the last 1-2 minutes of your shower ice cold
- Take an ice bath

- Run with less clothing if the weather is cold
- Run with more clothing if the weather is hot
- Spend time in the sauna. You can also exercise in the sauna
- Walk barefoot over rocks, in snow, on hot pavement
- If you drink alcohol, get up early and train after you have had a little too much to drink the night before
- Run short distances barefoot
- If you live in a cold climate, drive to work with the windows down

The possibilities are endless. Be creative. Do something every day that challenges your comfort level. And remember to smile while you are doing it! You will notice an exciting transformation as you do this. Initially, it might take a lot of mental focus or toughness to be able to do these things. As you progress however, you will simply accept these uncomfortable situations as normal and they won't feel nearly as uncomfortable.

The next piece of your mental training program is mental imagery, commonly referred to as visualization. We will talk about visualization to improve your running technique in the next chapter. The first part of visualization for your mental training program refers to imagining how you will respond when things do not go as planned. For example, imagine yourself feeling nauseous or feeling exhausted on a tough part of the race. Think about how you will respond. This works even better if you can find pictures or videos of tough parts of the race.

The more detail you have in your visualizations, the better. See yourself in these situations staying calm and moving forward. I find it helpful during these times to think about just putting one foot in front of the other...and yes, smiling! Focusing on your breath or repeating a mantra such as "one foot in front of the other", "easy day" or "keep moving" can be especially helpful when you want to quit. The purpose of this type of visualization is when these situations occur, you have "been there before" and you know how to handle them.

The other part of visualization for your mental training program is seeing yourself finishing the race. This is where it gets fun! When you visualize your finish, be as specific as you can. Find a picture of the finish line so you know exactly what it looks like. Who will be there when you finish? Do you have a pacer with you? The key piece is to feel what it's like to finish the race. Think about your emotions when you cross the finish line. This helps to create the certainty in your mind that you will finish the race. You have already experienced the emotion of finishing the race. This may seem a little "out there" or "woo woo" for some of you, but trust me it works. I remember training for the Hardrock 100 being on the stair climber going through a mental movie of what the finish was going to be like. Many times, I got choked up and teary eyed going through this process. I got chills and my entire body felt the positive emotions of finishing the race. This training made me even more certain I was going to finish.

The final piece of your mental training program is a mindful breathing practice. Those of you who already have a daily yoga or Qigong practice can stick with your current program. If you don't have a mindful breathing practice, we are going to keep it simple. Why is it important to have a mindful breathing practice? The purpose isn't just to help you relax in the moment. You may have heard of the sympathetic nervous system. This is the "fight or flight" nervous system that goes into overdrive when your brain senses danger or a threat. It evolved to respond to the stress of situations like an encounter with a saber tooth tiger. It responds to the stresses of everyday life the same way. Our brain responds to stress the same way regardless of how life-threatening the stress is. Stress from work, family, or finding time to train all activate your sympathetic nervous. This causes your body to release hormones such as cortisol and adrenaline. This is very useful if we are running from a saber tooth tiger. It is very harmful when it happens frequently in response to the stresses of everyday life. This process creates more inflammation in your body and can weaken your immune system. Simply put, the stress of everyday life weakens your body. Some of you may be thinking, "I don't feel stressed" or "I perform better when I'm stressed". Trust me, this is just as important as your physical training.

The purpose of this practice is to create resilience and train yourself not to go into "fight or flight" mode when there is no real danger. Mental stresses break down your body just like physical stress does. All stresses are cumulative. This means you may be able to get away with running hard and not managing your mental stress during your training. However, the stress of race day may be just enough to put you "over the edge". Do you ever wonder why some runners can log many long runs without a problem but have gastrointestinal (GI) issues at mile 10 on race day? Their body finally broke down due to the combined mental and physical stress they experienced during training. You may be familiar with Irritable Bowel Syndrome (IBS). The latest research shows IBS is due to stress. There is clearly a link between GI issues and stress. Your mindful breathing practice will also help you stay calm when things don't go as planned. You will be stressed during the race. If you want to give yourself the best chance of finishing your 100-mile race, you must include a mindful breathing practice as part of your training!

If you haven't done mindful breathing before, don't over complicate things. You don't need to sit for an hour without thinking about anything. Perform the following for 10 minutes daily. Sit in a comfortable position and slowly inhale and exhale through your nose. Try to focus on your breath coming in and going out your nose. It may also be helpful to think of or say a word such as "calm" or "peace" on the exhale. This will help you relax and prevent your mind from wandering. If you are new to a mindful practice, your mind will tend to think about other things. This is normal and is OK. If you notice yourself thinking about other things, simply bring your attention back to your breath. Don't get frustrated! Think of mindful breathing as a "practice". You will not be perfect while you are doing it. The purpose is to train yourself to better handle stress. You have stress even if you don't realize it. If 10 minutes is too much, start with 2 minutes or whatever time is manageable. You want to create a habit so it becomes part of your day.

Your mindful breathing practice will not only make you a better runner, but will help you out in many other areas of your life. I started the practice when I was in my early 40s and pre-hypertensive. After 6 months of mindful breathing, my blood pressure has remained normal. Trust the process and begin your practice.

Summary of your mental training program:

- Do something that makes you uncomfortable daily
- Mindful breathing or similar practice daily (10 minutes)
- Visualize how you will respond when things don't go as planned (5 minutes)
- Create a strong mental movie of you finishing the race. (5 minutes minimum)

Some runners find it easier to perform the visualization practices immediately after the mindful breathing. Do whatever works best for you.

How do you run strong and avoid injury?

It It is estimated between 65%-80% of runners get injured each year. Have you ever wondered why this number is so high? Many runners are told or assume running breaks down the body and causes knee or hip arthritis. While they may want to run forever, they think it's not realistic. Or maybe they want to keep running, but their healthcare provider tells them they should stop. "Running damages your knees" or "you're getting too old to run" are common things runners are told. If you train smart, there is no reason why you can't run forever.

When you consider the high injury rate, it makes you realize something is wrong with conventional running programs. What do you need to change with your training to minimize the risk for injury? Most running injuries are categorized as "overuse" type injuries. Plantar fasciitis, shin splints, Achilles tendinitis, "runner's knee", are common injuries sustained by runners. The high injury rates are due to training errors, muscle weakness, poor mobility (either from muscle tightness or joint stiffness), or running technique. Understanding the importance of these variables and improving them will help you run strong forever!

One reason runners get injured is training errors. This can include progressing your program too quickly, running too many miles, or not allowing yourself enough recovery time. It is important to remember that every tissue (muscle, tendon, bone, ligament) in your body is constantly remodeling itself. All tissues get stronger when you apply "controlled stress". Controlled is the keyword. Overstressing a tissue by running too many miles, poor running form, not being strong enough, not having good mobility, or not having enough recovery time can lead to tissue breakdown and injury. However, applying the right amount of stress will cause the tissue to remodel itself stronger. The right amount of stress will vary from runner to runner. It will also depend on factors such as your nutrition, sleep, and stress level.

You must also remember that stress is cumulative. This means you may be able to get away will high mileage weeks for months or even years, but eventually it will lead to injury. You also need to understand other impact activities such as plyometric strengthening or fitness classes that have lots of stepping or jumping also stress your tissues. It is the combined total of running, jumping, or any impact type exercise you need to be aware of when you consider how much you are stressing your tissues. It's not just running! Additionally, tissue weakens as we age. Many young runners can log high mileage weeks without a problem. However, the problem (and injury) comes when they continue with that type of training as they get older. We don't need to stop running as we get older. We need to train smarter. Smart training now will pay off down the road and you won't become another running statistic.

While running too much can contribute to injuries, there are other factors that are important to consider. Are you a strong runner? By strong, I don't mean are you a fast runner. Are your muscles strong enough to withstand running your desired weekly mileage? Look around at distance runners. Do they look like strong athletes? Most distance runners are weak. Weakness leads to injuries. It also leads to a breakdown in running form. You will get lazy when you are tired. Your muscles are designed to withstand the stress of running. However, when you fatigue, much of the stress of running is transferred to your joints causing injury. Compare how many runners look at the beginning of a long race to the end of the race. Why is it their form is typically much worse at the end? Muscle fatigue is a major reason. Of course, we all are fatigued at the end of a race and don't look nearly as good as we did at the beginning. However, the stronger you are, the better your performance will be and the more resilient you will be to injury.

A common misconception is running strengthens your muscles and you don't need to do additional strength training. Running can help improve your muscle endurance for running. However, you need to have enough muscle mass and strength first. This doesn't mean you need to be huge. You just need enough strength to match your running goals. Your strengthening program should be specific to running. This means your exercises should strengthen your muscles the way they are stressed during running. Think about what your muscles need to do every time your foot hits the ground. Many muscles (not just your hip or core muscles) need to react quickly without you thinking about it. This is a "motor program" that needs to happen automatically with each step you take. Your training should stress your muscles in a similar manner. Runners that are working on their strength tend to focus on their hip and core muscles. They will do exercises such as planks, crunches, "clamshells", or bridges. These exercises may help build a basic strength foundation, but they are not specific to running (or any other functional activity). These exercises isolate a group of muscles. However, our muscles do not function in isolation.

They need to work together...quickly! Holding a plank for 2 minutes doesn't train your muscles to work how they need to when you are running. Again, think about how your muscles need to respond each time your foot hits the ground. Think about where the forces of your foot hitting the ground are going to go if your muscles aren't trained to absorb the impact. That's right...your joints.

Most runners I know love to run. They want to spend as much of their training time running instead of working on strengthening. If this is you, you need to think about what exercises are going to "give you the most bang for your buck". No exercise is bad. However, if you only have 60 minutes a week for strength training, I wouldn't recommend spending any of that time doing crunches or planks. If you are a runner that loves to strength train, fantastic! You will be a much better runner with fewer injuries when you apply the training principles recommended in this book.

How is your running technique?

Much has been written about running technique with many different opinions. Unfortunately, the research doesn't give us a clear-cut answer on the best way to run. Running is a sport that requires skill to perform optimally. Just like any other sport, there are things you can do to improve your technique and make you a better runner. Some runners and coaches don't spend any time thinking about or training technique. This is a huge mistake. Many coaches think if the running form is working for that person and they haven't been injured, there is no need to change it. Just because you don't have an injury now doesn't mean you won't get injured down the road. How many runners do you know have had to stop running as they have gotten older due to an injury? You can run for years with poor technique, and never get injured. This doesn't make it right, however.

There are some runners who have beautiful technique without any instruction. Why is that? I think most of us know how to run at an early age. Watch any kid run across the grass barefoot. You won't see a lot of heel striking. It just doesn't feel good to land on your heel first. You likely will see a big smile on a kid having fun running landing on her forefoot (the balls of your feet)! If most of us know how to run as kids, what happens as we get older? Running shoes (more on running shoes in the next chapter), lack of strength and mobility, and lack of coaching are to blame.

Some running experts will argue most runners are heel strikers (even some elite runners) and the research is inconclusive if heel striking leads to injury.

Therefore, we shouldn't focus on how a runner lands. We need to recognize research has its limitations. We need to also consider what makes the most sense. Jump up and down landing on your heel compared to landing on the balls of your feet. What feels better? Obviously, it is much more natural to land on your forefoot (the balls of your feet). Your muscles and tendons are in a much better position to absorb shock with a forefoot landing. A runner may be able to run for years heel striking and never get injured. This doesn't mean it's the right way to run.

So how do you know if you have good running technique? Two key things to look for are a forefoot landing (your heel should gently kiss the ground immediately after your forefoot) and landing with your center of mass (chest/hips) over your foot. I recommend taking a video of you running to see how you run. I see many runners who think they are forefoot strikers. When we watch them run on video, they are landing heel first.

The most common error is landing with a heel strike with your foot in front of your center of mass. When you land with your foot in front of your center of mass (COM) your muscles need to work to slow you down until your COM catches up to your foot. Your knee will also be straighter in this position compared to landing with your foot under your COM. A straighter knee means more of the landing forces are transmitted to your joints instead of muscles. This stress is transmitted from your feet all the way up your body leading to injury.

There are a couple easy strategies that can clean up these common errors. Try to increase your cadence (steps per minute or the number of times each foot hits the ground) to 180. A higher cadence will typically result in more of a forefoot strike with your foot landing more under your center of mass. A higher cadence at a slower pace will usually mean you are taking shorter strides. The faster you run, the better a higher cadence will feel because your stride will feel more natural. Even if you typically run at a slower pace, it is good to practice running fast for 15-30 seconds several times during a run to help train the higher cadence. For optimal running performance and injury prevention, you want to minimize your foot contact time on the ground. It can help to be especially mindful about quickly pulling your foot up each time it hits the ground. Some runners find it helpful to think about running across hot coals or glass when trying to increase their cadence.

Another great strategy to improve your running technique is running barefoot on grass. The purpose isn't to change you to be a barefoot runner. You have nerve receptors in your foot and ankle that tell your brain where your foot is. These are called proprioceptors and are very important for balance and running performance. A running shoe limits the amount of information that travels to your brain because it places a barrier between your foot and the ground. When you run barefoot you get a much better sense of how your foot hits the ground. You will also be able to react quicker and increase your cadence because you will have less cushioning between your foot and the ground. This helps to train your muscles to react quickly each time your foot hits the ground. Practice running barefoot at varying speeds from a slow jog to a sprint with a high cadence. Running distances of 50-100 yards with a short break in between for 5-10 minutes, 1-2 days per week is enough. Be careful not to spend too much time running barefoot if you are used to running in shoes. Running barefoot does increase the stress on your plantar fascia and Achilles tendon so you must progress slowly. You will get injured if you don't gradually progress! However, as mentioned previously these tissues will get stronger with controlled stress. Incorporating barefoot training into your program will help strengthen the muscles in your feet, your plantar fascia, and Achilles tendon and reduce your injury risk if done appropriately.

What is the best running shoe for you?

Over the last few decades there has been many technological advances in shoe cushioning and support. Unfortunately, this has not resulted in a reduction in running injuries. The traditional running shoe prescription model (choosing a cushioned, stability, or motion control shoe based on "foot type") has led many to believe that too much pronation (foot rolling inward) is a bad thing that needs to be controlled. In addition, many believe if you have high arches you need more cushioning. We have also seen trends from extreme minimalist footwear (even barefoot) to extremely highly cushioned running shoes. This has led to much confusion among runners.

Our foot is a remarkable structure composed of numerous muscles, bones, ligaments, and tendons that are uniquely designed to adapt to the stress of running. The complex structure of the foot allows it to pronate (roll inward) and absorb impact when it strikes the ground. The foot then supinates (rolls outward) to create a rigid lever to help propel us forward.

Pronation is a normal movement of your foot that serves a very important purpose of shock absorption. If you use a rigid shoe or support to control pronation, you are limiting your foot's ability to help absorb shock. Your foot should be allowed to move as naturally as it can when it hits the ground. There is some thought that "excessive pronation" needs to be controlled with some type of support. You want to allow pronation to occur naturally and control it with your muscles in your foot, ankle, hip, and core. Strong muscles along with good foot and ankle mobility will help you absorb the impact of running and reduce your risk of injury. The rigid arch support found in many running shoes may weaken the muscles and tendons in the foot because your muscles do not need to work as much to control the foot. Think about if you have ever been in a cast. What happens to your muscles? They atrophy or get smaller. Muscles are supposed to be stressed. That is how they get stronger. While a rigid arch support is different than a cast, the concept is similar. The support is limiting the stress on your muscles. Controlled stress will strengthen your muscles while not causing injuries to your plantar fascia or Achilles tendon.

Some of you may be thinking, "I have arch supports and my feet feel better and I have no pain!". Arch supports may make you feel better and decrease pain. I have had many patients over the years tell me how great they feel with arch supports. Arch supports do the job your muscles, tendons, and ligaments are supposed to do. It is fine to use arch supports for a short period to help relieve your pain. However, if you want to run forever, it makes much more sense to strengthen your muscles so you don't need to rely on arch supports. A good analogy I use with patients is if someone has low back pain. With low back pain, common practice is not to have the patient wear a back brace that supports their back. Instead, they are encouraged to get stronger and maintain mobility. So why do some running experts and health care providers think it's a good idea to recommend an arch support that helps do the job your muscles should be doing and limits your foot's normal mobility?

At the other end of the shoe spectrum are cushioned running shoes. A heavily cushioned shoe leads to a decreased ability to "feel" the ground when your foot hits the ground. It is important to be able to feel the ground when your foot strikes the ground so your muscles can make minor adjustments to improve control and stability. To get this feedback in a cushioned shoe, the foot needs to land with more force than it would with a less cushioned shoe. Recent research has shown your landing forces are lowered with less cushioned shoes. A shoe with a lot of cushion also creates a more unstable surface. A more unstable surface causes more movement in your foot and ankle which can lead to injuries. Some of you may do balance training standing on cushioned and unstable surfaces. This is fine for training, but it doesn't make sense to run on a heavily cushioned unstable surface when you run.

So, what type of shoe is best for you? You should select a shoe that has the least amount of cushioning and support that feels good to you. You want your foot to move the way it was designed to move. Your strength, mobility, and how long you have been running in a more cushioned or supportive shoe will determine how much support and cushion you need. The type of running you do is also important to consider. You will want a little more cushioning if you are running roads versus a soft trail.

Transitioning to a minimalist shoe typically makes the most sense for most runners. This doesn't mean you need to run with just a thin rubber sole under your foot. A minimalist shoe is one that has less stability and cushioning compared to a traditional running shoe. There is also less difference between the heel and forefoot height. The heel is 12-15 mm higher than the forefoot in a traditional shoe compared to a 0-10 mm difference in a minimalist shoe. While the greater heel height in traditional shoes may reduce stress on the Achilles tendon, the reduced stress weakens the tendon over time. It also causes your calf muscles to become tight. Furthermore, the increased heel height also tends to promote more of a heel strike. A minimalist shoe allows your muscles to better control your foot motion and lets your feet feel the ground when running. This results in less impact and better control. It also tends to promote a more natural, more efficient running gait.

If you decide to transition to a minimalist shoe, it is important to do it gradually otherwise you could set yourself up for injury. Your muscles, especially the ones in your feet and your calf will work much harder in a minimalist shoe. Progressing slowly will allow your muscles, tendons, and ligaments time to adapt to the new stresses of a less supportive shoe.

Understanding common running injuries

What if you do everything right? You have good strength and mobility, you have good running technique, you are on top of your mental game, you wear the correct shoes...and yet...you still get injured. It makes sense with most injuries to have an active recovery. This means you can still be active, but you need to adjust your training program. This may include things such as changing what exercises you do or reducing your time or intensity exercising. An exception to this rule would be if you are overtrained. Unfortunately, this is becoming more common with ultra-runners because many runners run too many miles. If you are feeling excessively fatigued or tired or don't recover from your runs like you usually do, you could be overtrained. The sooner you back off, the better. Oftentimes, it makes sense to seek out the help of a functional medicine health care provider to help with your recovery. A functional medicine provider can help you figure out what nutritional imbalances may be contributing to your symptoms. Excessive running doesn't just cause orthopedic injuries. It can throw your whole body out of whack.

Runners more commonly suffer from injuries such as a tendonitis (Achilles or knee), plantar fasciitis, or other types of knee pain including "runner's knee" (pain underneath or around the kneecap) and IT band syndrome. Many of these injuries were once thought to be inflammatory. Any medical condition that ends in "-itis" means there is inflammation. A common treatment for these injuries commonly includes rest, ice, and anti-inflammatories such as ibuprofen. However, recent research has shown these injuries have very little if any inflammation once they become more chronic. Therefore, it makes no sense to treat them with ice and anti-inflammatory medication. Keep in mind that both ice and most anti-inflammatory medication may decrease your pain. There are small tears in the tendon or plantar fascia that weakens its structure. This contributes to the pain associated with these injuries. Because of this, it can be especially harmful to treat conditions such as plantar fasciitis with cortisone or other steroid injections. Steroids weaken tissue which can increase the risk of tissue rupture in tissue that is already weak. These injuries are more appropriately called a tendinopathy or plantar fasciopathy (instead of plantar fasciitis).

How should a tendinopathy or plantar fasciopathy be treated? The research shows tendons and the plantar fascia get stronger with strengthening exercises. Much of the research has focused on eccentric exercises, but it is not clear if eccentric is necessarily better than concentric strengthening. If you have a tendon injury, you need to stress it to stimulate your body to remodel the tendon stronger. As mentioned earlier, "controlled stress" is key. Too much stress can cause tissue breakdown.

Similar principles apply to "runner's knee". Too many times runners who have knee pain are advised to avoid squatting too deep or never let your knees go over your toes. While this strategy may help decrease your pain, the cartilage around your knees will get weaker if it is not progressively stressed. There is a common misconception that squatting deep or letting your knees go over your toes will damage your knees. It does not. If you have spent any time in Asian cultures, you have seen many elderly adults can easily hang out for long periods of time in a full squat position. The reason many Western adults can't fully squat keeping their heels on the ground is because most stop doing it as they grow up. Most all of us could fully squat when we were playing as a kid. As we get older, we have no reason to fully squat and we are often told we should avoid it. So, what happens? We lose the mobility and flexibility to squat and our knees become weaker making them vulnerable to injury. This cycle continues. Our knees hurt so we squat less which weakens the knees and causes pain. We tend to squat less and not go as deep because of the pain. And our knees continue to get weaker.

It is also worth mentioning stress fractures. Although uncommon with recreational runners, stress fractures can occur, especially with high mileage and progressing too quickly. The most common areas are the feet and shins but you can get them in the hip and low back as well. Your physical therapist will be able to help determine if a stress fracture is likely and possibly recommend further testing if necessary.

Any time you get injured, you should be evaluated by a qualified professional to help you figure out why you got injured. Only resting may help, but it is important to get to the root cause so injuries can be prevented in the future. As mentioned previously, running technique, muscle weakness, and limited mobility are common causes of running injuries. It is very common for other muscles to "shut down" or stop working when a runner gets injured. In other words, your muscles get weaker when you are injured. For example, research has shown the hip muscles shut down and become weaker with a sprained ankle. This is another way your brain tries to protect you. It causes other muscles to shut down to try and prevent you from doing any activity that might cause more damage. The muscle strength typically doesn't return even when the pain goes away. Therefore, it is important to specifically train the weakened muscles. If this weakness isn't addressed, you are more likely to get injured in the future.

Why all runners need to understand pain

All of us have experienced pain at some time in our lives. Maybe you hurt your back lifting something, sprained your ankle while running, or simply experienced neck pain from spending too much time at your computer. Pain is a necessary protective mechanism that serves as a warning signal that you might be doing damage. However, the amount of pain one experiences frequently does not correlate with the amount of tissue damage. Furthermore, pain can persist even after the injured tissue has fully healed. It is common to think of pain as an input to the brain. For example, if you notice a twinge in your knee on a run and you feel pain, you may think that pain travels to the brain to warn of possible danger. However, research has shown pain is an output from the brain and not input. When a tissue such as muscle, ligament or disc is overstressed the nerve fibers send "danger signals", not "pain signals" to the brain. Your brain takes this input along with input from your hormones, immune system, autonomic nervous system, and your thoughts, memories, and emotions to decide whether or not to "sound the alarm" and cause pain. Pain as defined by the International Association for the Study of Pain is an "unpleasant sensory and emotional experience, associated with actual or potential tissue damage, or described in terms of such damage". The key point is to remember pain is both a sensory and emotional experience.

Phantom limb pain provides a good example of how pain truly is output from the brain. Phantom limb pain is the experience of pain in a body part that does not exist. Seventy percent of people who have suffered an amputation experience a phantom limb.

These symptoms which can include itching, tingling or pain in the missing limb generally increase when the person becomes stressed. They may also increase when another person comes close to where the body part would have been. Although the body part no longer exists, the pain experienced is very real. This is because pain originates in the brain and spinal cord and not where the pain is felt. Though the body part no longer exists all the brain circuitry responsible for sensation and control of the body part remains and is fully functioning.

While acute pain is normal (such as that from an ankle sprain) and in most cases, helps protect us from doing more damage, persistent or chronic pain is a different story. In many cases of chronic pain, the damaged tissues have healed, but the pain persists. Like phantom limb pain, changes in the brain and spinal cord contribute to the vicious cycle of chronic pain. The nervous system becomes much more sensitive and pain is felt even when there is no damage to tissues such as your plantar fascia, tendons, and muscles. Some individuals with chronic pain experience an increase in pain even when they don't move, are under stress, or even just think about their pain. While it may seem this increase in pain occurs for no reason, it happens because your nervous system decides to pay closer attention to these now faulty danger signals and thus produce pain. For example, it is very common for runners with plantar fasciopathy (plantar fasciitis) to have pain walking barefoot. Walking barefoot does not cause damage to the plantar fascia in most cases. However, it can cause severe pain due to the sensitivity of the nervous system.

The good news is the changes to the nervous system are reversible and it is possible to dial down the nervous system's sensitivity to pain. The most effective treatment is one where you combine ways to decrease irritating signals coming in and maximize the incredible power of the brain to prevent these signals from becoming pain.

If your nervous system is ramped up from years of a persistent running injury, you need to "rewire" your nervous system. Remember our brain receives input from several sources to help determine if we will experience pain. For example, runners with plantar fasciopathy will receive "danger signals" from the foot. However, this signal alone does not dictate if they will experience pain. Our brain takes the "danger signal" from the foot along with several other inputs in determining whether or not to "sound the alarm" and cause pain. The brain then is the key to determining what stimulus is worthy of triggering pain. Factors such as stress, sleep loss, history of pain, and expectations of pain all increase the sensitivity of the brain to "danger signals". Furthermore, many runners are very much in tune with their bodies. If we have pain on a run, we try to figure out what we may be doing to cause the pain. Being aware of your body can serve you well in some cases. However, if you have persistent pain and you are continually analyzing why you are hurt, you are continuing to draw your brain's attention to the painful area. This will cause your brain "to pay more attention" to any danger signals coming up from the painful area. This makes it more likely for you to experience pain. I am not recommending ignoring pain. You just need to understand there is both a physical component to pain and an emotional (nervous system) component. This is true for all pain, not just chronic pain. For example, if I have a big race coming up in 3 weeks and I notice pain in my foot that gets worse during my run, I will likely be more concerned about this pain than if the race was 3 months away. Or maybe I have a friend who experienced similar pain and couldn't run for 6 months. These thoughts will create more stress in my nervous system. Increased stress makes my alarm system more sensitive and therefore I am more likely to experience pain even if I am not causing damage.

It is normal to think that pain means you are causing damage. However, it is more accurate to think of pain as a warning signal indicating you may be doing damage. In individuals with chronic pain the nervous system is hypersensitive and therefore will "sound the alarm" and cause pain when there is no damage. The first step in managing chronic pain and "rewiring your brain" is recognizing this and reassuring yourself that part of the reason for your pain is the increased sensitivity of the nervous system. The increased sensitivity can begin very soon after an acute injury. Understanding this can prevent acute injuries from becoming chronic injuries. Research has shown the more you understand about pain and how it works, the better you will do. Simple reassurance to yourself that you are not causing damage with a particular activity will dial down your nervous system's sensitivity. Obviously, there are cases when running will cause more damage such as a stress fracture or other more serious injury. A physical therapist who is an expert in pain can help you identify activities that may cause you pain, yet are not causing damage. Unfortunately, many healthcare providers don't have a thorough understanding of how pain works and don't educate patients on the importance of treating both the injured area and the ramped up nervous system.

Another technique to help "rewire the brain" is visualization. Many of you may be familiar with how athletes frequently visualize performing their sport as part of their training program. You may even do it. Visualization activates parts of the nervous system that are involved in the physical performance of the sport. This has been shown to improve performance. We can decrease pain with running by visualizing running feeling great! You must visualize the activity pain-free! Remember, history of pain with an activity and expecting pain with an activity provides input to your brain making it more likely you will experience pain. If running has caused pain previously, it is normal to expect it to cause pain again. Visualizing running without pain will dial down the part of the nervous system that "expects" or anticipates pain with running. This input over time will help with the "rewiring" process and decrease your pain.

It can be challenging to know if you are causing damage when you experience pain with running or if your nervous system is ramped up. This is when it can be helpful to work with a physical therapist who understands pain. Your therapist can help guide your progression. You need to still respect your pain even if it is not causing damage. Running through pain and ignoring it can oftentimes get your nervous system more ramped up increasing your pain. Therefore, it is important to gradually progress running at a rate that won't cause tissue damage and will allow your nervous system to recalibrate. I find it helpful to think of pain as a "yellow light". If you experience pain and it is reasonable to think you are not causing damage, reassure yourself you are OK. Thinking or saying to yourself "This is OK, I am not causing damage, my pain is real. My nervous system is just ramped up and will calm down" can be helpful. It doesn't need to be these exact words, but you need to reassure yourself you are not causing damage and you are safe to run. Remember, you feel pain when your brain perceives a threat. Your brain is perceiving running as a dangerous activity. This strategy isn't simply thinking positive or happy thoughts. You are giving your brain input that says it is OK to run. There is no need to sound the alarm and cause pain.

If you reassure yourself and your pain continues to get worse, you should back off. However, some stress to your tissue at the appropriate time will help your tissue get stronger. It is important to find the amount of running and other exercises that won't cause damage and won't get your pain flared up. Gradually progressing from that point will help your tissue get stronger and your nervous system calm down.

I use the reassurance strategy even though I don't have persistent pain. If I am on a run and feel a twinge, I will reassure myself I am OK. I think of it as the "yellow light". Oftentimes the pain goes away immediately. If it doesn't, I may take a few days off running to reduce the stress on the tissue. This strategy is especially important if you are a "type A" runner. This means if you feel a pain you immediately analyze why it happened. Thoughts such as "what did I do wrong" are common. If running is a big part of your life you can easily get your pain ramped up by your thoughts. "What if I can't do that race" or "I can't take time off running" are stressful thoughts. Stress makes it more likely to experience pain. Of course, it makes sense to understand why you have pain. Just don't overdo it!

Your nutrition and hydration plan

The optimal nutrition plan will depend on race conditions and will vary among runners. The best nutritional plan is the one that works for you. It is also one that you have practiced during your training runs. Never try anything new on race day! Try keeping the food you eat during an ultramarathon like the food you normally eat. Remember your body and gut are already going to be stressed. Try to minimize additional stress by eating like you normally do as much as possible. A general guideline is to eat between 150-300 calories per hour. Start eating early in the race and eat at regular intervals. Setting your watch to remind you to eat every 15-30 minutes will help keep you on track. Many times, it can be difficult to keep eating, especially racing at a higher altitude. I recommend eating whatever tastes good even if it is not the most nutritious food. You need calories to keep you going! Figure out what combination of gels, sports drinks, and real food work best for you. The key thing is for you to practice your nutrition plan during your training. It can also be helpful to have some caffeine during the race. Caffeine has been shown to decrease the rate of perceived exertion (RPE). This means you won't feel as tired or fatigued as you would if you didn't have caffeine. Many races will have caffeinated soda at aid stations. You can also find some gels with caffeine. My personal favorite however, is chocolate covered espresso beans!

Your fluid and electrolyte intake will also vary greatly depending on the race conditions. 12-20 ounces of fluid per hour is a good place to start. You will also want to include electrolytes either through a sports drink or capsule. Drinking too much water without additional electrolytes can lead to a dangerous condition called hyponatremia. If you want to be a little more precise with figuring out how much fluid you need, weigh yourself naked before an hour-long run. Run for an hour in race conditions without consuming anything. Dry the sweat off and weigh yourself again. This can help estimate the amount of fluid you lose in an hour. Start your hydration early in the race so you don't become dehydrated. A 3% loss in body weight due to dehydration can decrease your performance by 15%. Ideally, you should consume plenty of water every day (clear urine is a good indicator you are). However, it is especially important the week of the race to be sure you start the race fully hydrated.

Your training plan

Phase I (0-3 months)

This training plan is designed for runners who have never run an ultramarathon before and those who have but are looking for ways to improve their performance and not get injured. Phase I is the foundational phase of your running season. You need a strong foundation if you expect to have a successful running season. You will notice the amount of running I recommend is considerably less than what others may recommend. I also include upper body strengthening in the training program. I truly believe all of us can run forever. My passion is helping runners understand the best way to do this. If all you do is run, you will eventually get injured (if you haven't already) and your running career will be cut short. Excessive running will put you at risk for orthopedic injuries regardless of how strong you are. Hip and knee arthritis are common injuries that shorten a runner's career. So, what is excessive? Recent research has shown running greater than 57 miles per week increases the risk of getting knee and hip arthritis. However, running less than 57 miles per week reduces your risk for arthritis compared to people who don't run. Like many things in life, a moderate amount of running is good for us! This program is meant to be a simple guide to running an ultramarathon and keep you running injury free forever. Many runners I talk to feel they must run high mileage to be able to run an ultramarathon. That is not the case. It may be true you could run a faster ultra with more training. And maybe it is worth it to you. However, I would encourage you to take a long-term approach to your training. Be strong and mobile, run moderate distances, and you will be able to run forever!

If you already have a solid running base, feel free to adjust the times or distances of your runs during the initial phase of your training. Additionally, think of this phase as your offseason from running. Every runner should have an offseason. This doesn't mean you can't run during this time. It means you should cut back to 2 easy runs per week. Your focus during your offseason should be on allowing your body to recover from an intense season of running and getting stronger. You can still cross train with low impact exercises. Strength is hugely important if you want to run as well as you can forever while minimizing your risk of injury. As mentioned previously, you get weaker and lose muscle power as you age. This usually begins to happen in your 30s. You may not notice it because it happens very slowly and "sneaks up on you". You may even be able to continue running your typical distances and pace as you lose power and muscle mass. However, it will eventually catch up with you. You need to strength train! While you can do some strength training during your running season, it will be limited. It will be too much for you to do the strength training required and continue running more than 2 days per week.

The training recommendations in this book are very general and follow the 80-20 principle. One of my main purposes for writing this book is because you can finish an ultra-marathon with less training than you probably think. I wrote this book for runners who want to complete an ultra-marathon, but want to do it in the most efficient way with the least amount of training. I also think we sometimes make things more complicated than they need to be. Additionally, ultra-runners tend to overtrain and do too much running. I like to keep things simple and choose the most effective and efficient exercise program I can to accomplish my goal. I understand some runners will want to do more than what I recommend. It is fine to make some additions to the training program if you follow the principles outlined in this book.

During phase I of your training program, you will focus on building a running base (if you do not already have one), improving your running technique, getting stronger, and improving your mobility. It will include 2 days of easy running, 1 day of strength training with an emphasis on legs, 1 day of strength training with an emphasis on upper body, and 1 day of plyometric type exercises. You may be asking "what about core exercise?" Of course, you need to have a strong core for running. However, the fitness industry has led many to believe the best way to work your core muscles is to work them in isolation. Common exercises such as crunches or planks are not bad exercises, but they isolate your abdominal and back muscles. The problem with this is we don't function in running or life by using our muscles in isolation. Your core muscles need to work with many other muscles very quickly and precisely to optimize your run performance. Therefore, it makes the most sense to train your muscles in a way that is similar to how they function when you run. Every exercise in this program strengthens your core along with many other muscles. Common core exercises are not included because they are typically not the best exercises for runners to do.

Phase I is also the time to work on your focus and concentration with your running technique and strength training. Too many times I see athletes simply going through the motions when they do their strength training. They may spend 2 hours in the gym, but the quality isn't there. It is important to focus on the muscles you are training with each exercise. Similarly, many runners don't think about their technique while running. I understand running can be great for stress relief and it is fine to "zone out" and not think about anything during your runs. However, you need to spend part of your time running focused on your technique.

The running recommendations I give are very general and you don't need any special equipment such as a heart rate monitor or other high-tech devices. However, these devices can be a very helpful to keep your training more specific and provide feedback on your progression. There are also some great tools that give you feedback on your running cadence and vertical displacement (how much you bounce up and down when you run). If you want more guidance on the exact pace you should be running during a particular workout the Jack Daniels' Running VDOT Calculator is a great free tool that can be found at runsmartproject.com/calculator.

For phase I, run 2 days per week at an easy pace for 30-45 minutes. An easy pace is defined as being able to easily maintain a conversation during your run. If you haven't run before or if it has been a while, it is best to gradually begin running by alternating walking and running. Begin by alternating walking and running each minute for 30 minutes. Gradually increase your time running over the next 12 weeks. You should be running an easy pace for a straight 30-45 minutes by the end of this phase.

This is also the time to work on your running technique. Run barefoot on grass 5 minutes before your easy runs (or stop at a park or golf course during your run). Remember to vary your speed and focus on a high cadence. Think of running with light, quick steps. Be sure to "check in" with your technique throughout your run.

Your Mobility Program

When I ask most runners about their flexibility or mobility program, many are embarrassed to say either they don't have one or maybe they spend 2 minutes stretching before or after a run. I get it. You are a runner and you like to run! We all have a limited amount of time to train. If you have 30 minutes to train, you want to run. You don't want to spend 20 minutes stretching and 10 minutes running. The good news is you don't have to. Yes, in a perfect world you might spend 20 minutes or more a couple days per week working on your mobility. Mobility work however, is especially important as we get older. Like everything else in this book, I am going to keep your mobility training simple and give you the two most important mobility exercises to work on. The best part is this will only take 4 minutes per week... 2 minutes two days per week. Of course, you can do more. However, remember we are looking for the most benefit with the least amount of time.

It is most important for runners to have good ankle, knee, and hip mobility. This can be accomplished with two simple exercises. They are a full squat with your feet and knees together and a "twisting" squat. You can find videos of these exercises at the Stronger Over Forty YouTube channel. You may be thinking squats are for strength.

They are great for strength, but they can also be great for mobility. When runners think of flexibility, many think of muscle stretching being held for several seconds to several minutes. Mobility exercises are more dynamic in nature (you will perform continuous repetitions instead of holding for a period) and not only improve muscle "flexibility", but they also help to improve joint mobility and provide nutrition to your joints. The more nutrition your joints get, the stronger they will be. Motion is lotion!

You may be asking, "what about hamstring stretching?" or you may have been told, "you have tight hamstrings and need to stretch them". For whatever reason, runners are commonly told they should stretch their hamstrings. If you are a ballet dancer, gymnast, or rock climber hamstring flexibility can be very helpful for your sports performance. For runners, it is not as important as you may think. You don't need to be able to touch your toes to be a good runner. You need to have strong hamstrings because your hamstrings work hard when you are running. The strength and mobility work in this program will give you the hamstring flexibility you need.

Your Leg and Core Strength Training Program

Your leg and core strength training routine should include the following and can be performed 1 day per week:

- Single leg squat
- Single leg deadlift
- Goblet squat

- Deadlift or Kettlebell swing (If kettlebell swings are new to you, I recommend perfecting your deadlift technique before your move on to kettlebell swings)

Videos of these exercises can be found at the Stronger Over Forty YouTube channel. There is no magic number for how many sets or repetitions you need to do. However, your muscles should be tired and you should feel fatigued when you are done. Remember to focus on the muscles you are training. Don't just go through the motions! I recommend 3 sets of 6-12 repetitions unless you are new to strength training. If you have not done any strength training, begin with 3 sets of 10 with the single leg deadlift and single leg mini squat. Additionally, perform the goblet squat without any weight. If you are not used to doing a full squat or if it causes you pain, reduce the depth of your squat so it is pain-free. As you get stronger, you should be able to go deeper. Contrary to what you may have been told or read, it is completely fine to do a full squat. It will not damage your knees. Additionally, many clients I work with have been told to never let their knees go over or in front of their feet. This is completely safe as well. Unfortunately, many runners will get pain with a squat. This may be related to running or the typical American lifestyle where we don't need to squat with our activities throughout the day. Runners are frequently told to avoid squatting or don't go as deep if they do squat. The problem with this advice is your knees get stronger with "controlled stress" just like every other tissue in your body. If you avoid a full squat, not only will your muscles be weaker, but your knees will get weaker as well. However, it is very important to progress slowly and listen to your body. Your body needs time to adapt to any new stress, otherwise you will get injured.

If you are like many runners and do not want to go to the gym, this program can be easily performed at home with a few kettlebells. You should be able to complete it in about 30 minutes.

The exercises above are the minimum recommendations that can be done with little time and significantly improve your running. However, if you want to spend more time strength training, feel free to add other exercises. I recommend keeping your exercises "functional" and include variations of squats, lunges, and deadlifts. These exercises not only strengthen your legs but are great core exercises as well. Functional means the exercises more closely simulate what you need to do in life. Spending time on an exercise machine does not. Most machines isolate one movement or muscle group and require the user to sit. The machine is keeping you and the weight stable. You want your muscles to do the work to keep you and the weight stable and controlled.

Your Upper Body and Core Strength Training Program

Many runners don't realize the importance of upper body strength training. The reality is every part of your body is connected. Every part of your body needs to be able to work together for optimal running performance. Think of your body as a chain. Every link in that chain needs to work as one unit to help absorb the shock of running and keep you moving forward in the most efficient manner possible. Weakness in any part of the chain will limit your run performance and increase your risk of injury. Don't neglect upper body strength training. This doesn't mean you need to spend hours per week working on upper body strength. Keep it simple. You only need to focus on push-ups and pull-ups. Pull-ups can be assisted either with a machine or resisted band if needed. Push-ups and pull-ups are two great exercises that work all your upper body muscles including your core. Don't be concerned with how many reps you do. Focus more on the quality of the movement. You can find videos of both exercises at the Stronger Over Forty YouTube channel.

Your Dynamic Training Program

Your dynamic exercise program will also be performed 1 day per week. This program includes quick, jumping and hopping type exercises to more closely simulate what your muscles need to do when you run. Think about what needs to happen each time your foot hits the ground with running. Lots of muscles from your feet all the way up to your neck need to react quickly without you even thinking about it. Your muscles need to react to your foot hitting the ground. This means they need to be able to absorb the shock of your foot hitting the ground and quickly propel your forward. Additionally, as we get older we lose power or explosiveness in our muscles. This is important to maintain a light, springy feeling when you run. It is also critical if you want to be a good downhill runner. Your muscles need to react very quickly with each step running down a technical trail. Exercises that require you to jump and be quick helps to train the quick response and strength needed to perform your best and be injury free.

Your dynamic exercise program can be found at the Stronger Over Forty YouTube channel and includes the following:

- Side shuffle, carioca, and skipping warm-up
- Jump rope warm-up (simulate jumping rope if you don't have a jump rope)
- Power skips
- 4 Square jumps/hop (with stick and quick)
- Squat jumps
- Depth jumps (advanced exercise- work up to this if dynamic training is new to you)
- Tuck jumps (advanced exercise- work up to this if dynamic training is new to you)

The amount of these exercises you do will depend on your current fitness level and if you have been doing similar exercises. You will get injured if you progress too quickly. If you are new to this type of training, spend 3-5 minutes on the warm up exercises followed by 1 of the other exercises performed at 50% of what you feel like you could maximally do. Add 1 exercise and gradually increase the intensity over the next several weeks. Obviously, dynamic exercises will put more stress on your muscles, joints, and tendons. That is why you can't do a lot of dynamic training during your season. It would be too much to combine this program with running several days per week. As with any other exercise gradually progress and perform the exercises slower to give your body time to adapt. It is also a good idea to take the next day off to give your body time to recover. At a minimum, avoid impact exercise the day after your dynamic training.

I included the option of a sauna or ice bath on your rest days. These are not only great recovery tools, but can be used to work on your mental training as well.

Summary of Phase I (Mental Performance Training Program also performed most days of the week)

Day 1	Day 2	Day 3	Day 4	Day 5	Day 6	Day 7
Easy run	Mobility and dynamic training	Rest, sauna, or ice bath	Easy run	Mobility and lower body strength training	Rest, sauna, or ice bath	Upper body strength training. Cardio cross-train (optional)

Phase II (3-6 months)

By phase II, you should be feeling strong and have a solid running foundation. You are probably anxious to ramp up your running as well! During phase II you will increase your number of days running to 4 with 1 of those being a longer run and 1 being higher intensity. 2 of your runs will be 45-60 minutes at an easy pace. Your long run will be similar to your race pace. Your long runs should also be run on similar terrain to that of your planned ultra. If you are running an ultra on a trail with elevation change, you will likely power hike the climbs. Your long runs should include climbs and you should power hike them just like you will do on race day. Except for distance, your training runs should include much of the same conditions you will experience during the race. This includes visualizing parts of your race and loving every minute of it. Remember to intentionally make yourself uncomfortable during your training runs. Examples include running sleep deprived, running with wet shoes, and running with less clothing if it is cold. You need to train yourself to smile and embrace adversity. Begin to fine-tune your nutrition and hydration plan during your long runs as well.

Your first long run can be 90 minutes at an easy pace. You can gradually increase your time on your feet over the next several months. Notice how its "time on your feet" not "running". Some people don't realize most competitors in an ultra do not run the whole race. This is why many runners think it is necessary to run lots of miles in order to complete an ultra. You don't need to run lots of miles and even your long runs don't need to be as far as you may think. What is important is spending a lot of time on your feet. My longest training run prior to my first ultra, the Leadville 100, was around 28 miles. That "run" took me 6 or 7 hours because it was in the mountains simulating the exact conditions I was going to encounter during the race. I used a similar strategy to train for the Hardrock 100. The Hardrock 100 has 33,050 feet of elevation gain and 33,050 feet of elevation loss. The cut off time is 48 hours to finish the race. My total distance for one training run never exceeded 30 miles. My total weekly mileage never exceeded 60. However, my training was very specific to the race course and I spent a lot of time on my feet. It included lots of power hiking climbs and running easy on the descents and flats.

My point is to dispel the myth that you need to run a lot of miles if you want to run an ultra. Yes, you may be able to run a faster time with more training, but what is the cost? If your goal is like mine was (to complete a 100-mile race and continue to run forever), it might be worth a little slower time if it means you will be more likely to run forever, injury free.

As you progress your long runs leading up to the race, I recommend your weekly mileage not exceed 60. Remember, the research I referred to previously. Exceeding 57 miles is when your risk for knee and hip arthritis increases. Obviously, every runner is different and some may be able to run higher mileage. However, keep 60 miles in mind as you plan your weekly runs.

By now you should have a good understanding of how fast your easy runs should be and how to plan your long runs so they most closely simulate race conditions. Let's move on to your high-intensity day! How can you get the benefits of interval training with less time? Recently, a group of exercise physiologists in Denmark set out to determine if there was a way to reap the benefits of interval training, but in a less painful, less time-consuming manner. They came up with the 10-20-30 workout. The concept is simple. Jog for 30 seconds, run your normal pace for 20 seconds, and sprint for 10 seconds- then repeat four times. The researchers compared two groups of runners. One group continued their normal running routine while the second group replaced two of their three weekly workouts with the 10-20-30 workout. The 10-20-30 workout was repeated four times and was followed by a 2-minute recovery jog. This cycle was repeated two more times for a total run time of 16 minutes. At the end of the 8-week training program, the runners in the interval group improved their 5K times by an average of 38 seconds. Additionally, most runners also improved their blood pressure and cholesterol levels. The control group had no improvements in these measures. Although the interval group ran at a higher intensity, they reduced their mileage by 50%! Your high-intensity day should be similar to the 10-20-30 program.

Summary of Phase II (Mental Performance Training Program also performed most days of the week)

Day 1	Day 2	Day 3	Day 4	Day5	Day 6	Day 7
Long run	Rest, sauna or ice bath	Easy run	10-20-30 run	Rest, sauna, or ice bath	Easy run	Rest, sauna, or ice bath

Easy cross training can be performed on 1 of your rest days

You can also continue your upper body focused strength training from phase I

Phase III (6-9 months)

The physical training of phase III is the same as phase II. You will continue to increase your long runs, but remember to keep your weekly mileage less than 60 miles. However, you need to ramp up the intensity of your mental training during phase III. This means every long run should include visualizing yourself crossing the finish line. What are your emotions when you cross the finish line? How will it feel? Who will be there? What will your thoughts be when you finish? Ideally, you should train on the race course. If that is not possible, find pictures of the race course online. Implant them in your mind. Visualize the race course as you train. If you know that a certain part of the course is particularly difficult, imagine that part during your training. How will you feel? If it gets challenging, what will you do? What if you feel nauseous and start to vomit? How will you respond? What if it rains and you are without your jacket? Will you be mentally strong? Rehearse these scenarios in your mind during your training. Be as vivid as you can. If it happens on race day, you have already been there. There is no need to panic. Continue the race as planned knowing it will get better. Remember, you may feel like crap multiple times throughout the race and want to quit. The runners who smile and work through these times are the ones who finish. The rest DNF.

Summary of Phase III (Mental Training Program also performed most days of the week)

Day 1	Day 2	Day 3	Day 4	Day 5	Day 6	Day 7
Long run	Rest, sauna, or ice bath	Easy run	10-20-30 run	Rest, sauna, or ice bath	Easy run	Rest, sauna, or ice bath

Easy cross training can be performed on 1 of your rest days

You can also continue your upper body focused strength training from phase I

Final recommendations

How should you choose your race? Many runners I talk to who have a goal of running a 100-mile race feel they need to gradually work their way up to running a 100-mile race. They plan to run a 50K, then a 50 miler, then maybe a 100K, and finally a 100 miler. This is fine, but not necessary. If you train properly, there is no need to work up to a 100-mile race. My longest distance prior to running the Leadville 100 was a marathon. Get over any mental block you have about running 100 miles and do it!

When deciding which race to do, I recommend choosing one with lots of elevation gain. It is expected that you will hike a lot during the climbs. While you may suffer on some of the climbs because you are "sucking air", it is good to give your body a break from the constant impact of running. Regardless of whether you are training or racing, variety is good. Changing your speed and terrain will put different stresses on your body. It is also good psychologically. There is nothing like reaching the top of a climb and being able to "let it go" and fly down the trail!

Depending on the distance, some races will allow you to have a crew to transport your extra gear and a pacer after the first 50 miles. Otherwise, they will transport drop bags for you to various points along the course. If you have a pacer, be sure to communicate ahead of time how to best keep you motivated. Your mood will change when you are tired, cold, and want to quit. It will help you out tremendously if your pacer knows the right "buttons to push" to keep you going. My crew and pacers were a huge reason for me finishing my 100-mile races. My crew and pacers travelled several hours and gave up their weekends to help me finish a race. This gave me additional motivation not to let them down and quit.

Finally, let's talk about tapering. Your longest run and training weeks should be 3 weeks out from your race day. Reduce your mileage each week so the week before the race your longest run is 5-7 easy miles at most. My recommendation is to take the week off before the race. Your training is done at this point. An extra few days of running isn't going to give you much benefit. This also allows your body to more completely recover from any nagging injuries you have been pushing through. However, some runners psychologically "need to run" for a few days the week of the race. This is fine. Just keep the miles low and the pace slow.

Regardless of your running background, you should feel confident by now you can finish a 50 or 100-mile race. You control 95% of what determines whether or not you finish the race. The other 5% may include things such as lightning at high altitude races or acute sickness. Those are pretty good odds! Keep running strong!

Thank You

Before you go, I'd like to say "thank you" for purchasing this guide. I truly hope it has met your expectations and wish you the best wherever ultra running takes you! Find me on Facebook *@runstrongeroverforty* and let me know how your training goes!

If you have liked what you have read, it would mean a lot to me if you would please take a moment to leave a review for this book on Amazon.

I truly appreciate it.

Printed in Great Britain
by Amazon